Ouanassa Hamouda
Nabila Kalla
Khouloud Zemmouri

Osteo-muscular hydatidosis

Ouanassa Hamouda
Nabila Kalla
Khouloud Zemmouri

Osteo-muscular hydatidosis

ScienciaScripts

Imprint

Cover image: www.ingimage.com

This book is a translation from the original published under ISBN 978-620-6-72531-2.

Publisher:
Sciencia Scripts
is a trademark of
Dodo Books Indian Ocean Ltd. and OmniScriptum S.R.L publishing group

120 High Road, East Finchley, London, N2 9ED, United Kingdom
Str. Armeneasca 28/1, office 1, Chisinau MD-2012, Republic of Moldova, Europe
Printed at: see last page
ISBN: 978-620-8-20645-1

TABLE OF CONTENTS

INTRODUCTION

Hydatid cyst is a cosmopolitan parasitic disease. Despite the establishment of extensive prevention programmes, the disease is still rife in the Maghreb countries. It occurs mainly in sheep-breeding regions, and is still endemic in Algeria. Anthropozoonosis is a public health problem, threatening patients' vital prognosis because of the complications that can arise, as well as causing considerable economic losses **[1-3].**

The taenia Echinococcus granulosus is the causative agent of hydatid diseases. Its biological cycle comprises a definitive host, essentially the dog, and an intermediate host, mainly the sheep. As an accidental host, humans become infected via the digestive tract **[1].**

This infectious disease spares no organ. It most often affects the liver **[4]** following migration of the parasite through the portal venous system. If it manages to cross the hepatic filter, it is usually retained by the pulmonary capillaries, and if both the hepatic and pulmonary filters are crossed, the parasite can be captured by other organs such as the brain, heart, kidney, muscles and bones.Involvement of bone tissue is unusual. In this organ, the parasite evolves over 12 to 18 months to form the hydatid cyst, creating a multi-vesicular infiltration that destroys the bone **[5].** Clinically, the condition is generally asymptomatic, and may be revealed by suppuration or fistulisation, or discovered incidentally on imaging **[6].**

The muscular location of hydatid cysts is exceptional and slow to develop. It is important to consider this diagnosis, particularly in patients from endemic countries **[7].**Treatment is essentially surgical. It depends on the stage of the disease and, in particular, its location **[8].**

Prophylaxis is the main tool that needs to be put in place to interrupt the parasite cycle **[1].** Hydatidosis is an endemic disease in our country. Certain rituals practised within the Muslim community, such as the sacrifice of sheep during the Eid Al-Adha festival, contribute to the maintenance of the parasite cycle of the taenia Echinococcus granulosus. Our work concerns a retrospective study of osteo-muscular hydatidosis treated in the orthopaedics and traumatology department of the Benflis Touhami university hospital in Batna, over a period of 10 years, from January 2012 to December 2022. The main aim of this study is to fill the gap in data on the epidemiological profile of osteo-muscular hydatidosis in the Batna region.The secondary aim of our work is to highlight the risk and prognostic factors for hydatid cysts of bone and muscle.

PART I
THEORY

CHAPTER I

1. Bone system

1.1. General

The human skeleton is made up of two main parts:

• Appendicular skeleton (the bones of the girdle), i.e. the bones of the limb skeleton, including those forming the pelvic and pectoral (shoulder) girdles.
• Axial skeleton: comprising all the bones of the head of the skull, the neck (hyoid bone and cervical vertebrae) and the trunk (ribs, sternum, vertebrae and sacrum).

Bone is a highly specialised connective tissue with important functions:

✓ It contributes to the body's rigidity and protects the vital organs.

✓ Plays a mechanical role as a movement structure.

✓ Has a physiological role in the storage of minerals (calcium), as well as in haematopoiesis (production of blood cells via the bone marrow contained in many bones).

1.2. Anatomy of the bone

The bone structure that supports the human body is made up of bone and cartilage, which is a semi-solid, elastic form that gives some flexibility to certain skeletal structures (for example, the costal cartilage that connects the ribs to the sternum, and articular cartilage).

Cartilage has no vessels, so oxygenation of the chondrocytes is by diffusion. The proportion of cartilage in the skeleton remains small in adults.

The outer part of the bone is covered by a tissue called the periosteum, which is associated with the perichondrium, the tissue covering the cartilage. They contribute to the nutrition of the external parts of the skeletal tissues, and also provide insertion points for tendons and ligaments.

Depending on its density, bone tissue can take two forms:

- Compact bone tissue that gives bone its strength.
- Spongy bone tissue; within which haematopoiesis takes place.

Bones are linked together by joints, and unlike cartilage, bone tissue is richly vascularised and innervated.

For classification purposes, bones are divided into four categories:

- **Long bones**: are tubular (for example, the humerus in the arm). Their surfaces have prominences (crests and tubercles, ridges) forming a means of support, to ensure a strong muscular anchorage **[9].**

The structure of the long bones is made up of three parts:

✓ The diaphysis: formed by compact bone tissue, hollowed out by the medullary cavity occupied by the bone marrow.

✓ The epiphysis: formed by cancellous bone tissue.

✓ The metaphysis: this is the region in which the conjugation cartilage is found, and is the site of chondrocyte proliferation, enabling growth in length, as well as the site of enchondral ossification, the process by which bone replaces cartilage **[10].**

- **Short bones**: more or less cuboid in shape, found particularly in the ankle and wrist.
- **Flat bones**: generally play a role in protecting vital organs (for example, the flat bone in the vault of the skull, which protects the brain).
- **Irregular bones:** come in various forms, for example facial bones.
- **Sesamoid bones**: bones inserted inside certain tendons to protect them from excessive friction (e.g. the patella) **[9].**

1.3. Physiology of bone tissue

Bone tissue is a living thing that is constantly changing. This dynamic process allows the bone to renew itself, ensuring its strength and flexibility, and is closely regulated by a set of bone cells, minerals and hormones.

1.3.1. Bone tissue cells

Osteoblasts: osteoblastic cells are a heterogeneous group of cells of mesenchymal origin, including mature osteoblasts, osteocytes and border cells, with various functions. Mature osteoblasts are responsible for the formation of the extracellular matrix and the synthesis of type 1 collagen, glycosaminoglycans and other non-collagenous proteins **[11].**

Osteocytes: osteocytic cells are derived from osteoblasts and have metabolic activity. They are found embedded in the periosteocyte lacunae and may be involved both in the secondary formation of the calcified organic matrix and in its resorption.

Border cells: these are flattened, elongated cells located between the surface of the bone tissue (and its thin layer of osteoid tissue) and the haematopoietic tissue of the bone marrow. They may be involved in the preparation mechanism for remodelling **[10].**

Osteoclasts: these are giant cells with multiple nuclei of haematopoietic origin **[11].** They are responsible for the resorption of bone tissue **[10].**

1.3.2. The hormones

Parathyroid hormone PTH: this hormone is synthesised in the parathyroid gland in the form of an inactive precursor. It mobilises reserves and increases bone resorption. A drop in blood calcium levels activates its synthesis.

At renal level, it increases calcium reabsorption and reduces phosphate reabsorption, making it a hypercalcaemic and hypophosphataemic hormone.

1,25-Dihydroxycholecalciferol (vitamin D): plays a role in :

- Digestive; by increasing the digestive absorption of calcium and phosphate.
- Bone; where it stimulates osteoclastic bone resorption and promotes bone formation.
- Renal; in synergy with PTH, it increases tubular absorption (distal convoluted tubule) of calcium (and is therefore hypercalcaemic).

Vitamin D may play a role in regulating parathyroid hyperplasia in hyperparathyroidism, by exerting a negative feedback effect on PTH synthesis **[12].**

Calcitonin: a hormone involved in directly inhibiting the activity of osteoclasts (cells responsible for bone resorption).

Oestrogens: estradiol acts on osteoblastic cells, stimulating their proliferation, and on collagen, increasing its synthesis.

Bone remodelling takes place in four phases: the resorption phase, the intermediate phase, the formation phase and the quiescence phase.

This process is modulated by a group of cells, in particular osteoclasts (cells responsible for resorbing the mineralised matrix), which multiply and fuse with precursor cells. These cells are then attracted by chemotaxis to the site of bone resorption, where they anchor themselves by creating lacunae.

Once the process is complete, the osteoclasts will detach themselves from the bone surface, and information signals are sent out to trigger the bone formation phase. At the same time, during this phase (the intermediate phase), the areas that have not been resorbed by the osteoclasts are taken over by other cells responsible for eroding the irregularities in the calcified matrix that have not been resorbed.

The formation phase is ensured by the intervention of osteoblastic cells, which migrate to the resorption space and begin to produce and form a deposit of organic matrix, forming osteoid tissue.Finally, the bone surface remains inactive or quiescent until another remodelling cycle occurs **[11].**

2. General characteristics of muscular elements

Muscle is a contractile tissue that plays an essential role in movement via the joints **[13].**

2.1. Muscle structure

❖ Morphological aspect

There are two main types of muscle: striated and smooth.

✓ Striated muscles

The human body has 637 striated muscles. They are innervated by the cerebrospinal nervous system, and their contraction is voluntary. Each striated muscle consists of a middle part, a fleshy body and two extremities through which it is inserted.

Based on the shape of the fleshy body, a distinction is made between :

- Long muscles: the fleshy body is fusiform, ending in one or more tendons at each end. Sometimes, a muscle has two fleshy bodies, combined by an intermediate tendon.
- Flat muscles: the fleshy body is flat and wide, and the muscle fibres are inserted directly onto a large surface.
- Short muscles: the fleshy body is short and the muscle fibres are directly attached.
- Ring muscles: characterised by their circular shape. It is called an orbicular muscle if it surrounds a natural orifice, or a hollow viscus, in which case it is called a sphincter.

✓ Smooth muscles

Also known as involuntary muscles, because their contraction is controlled by the vegetative system. They are usually small and colourless.

❖ Histological study

The muscle fibre is a cell composed of a cytoplasm, known as the sarcoplasm, containing myofibrils, bounded by the sarcolemma.

✓ The striated muscle fibre

It is a very large cell, with each myofibril made up of a regular succession of light bands or I bands, and dark bands or A bands.

The histology of striated muscle fibre is characterised by double striation, longitudinal and transverse, due to the myofibrils and the alternation of light and dark bands, giving it its striated appearance.

✓ The smooth muscle fibre

It is smaller than striated muscle fibre. It has a sarcoplasm devoid of myoglobin, a single nucleus, unlike striated fibre which has many nuclei, and a cytoplasm containing homogeneous myofibrils, devoid of any striation.

2.2. Muscle physiology

Excitability, contractility, elasticity and tonicity are the main properties of striated and smooth muscles, although the contraction of the latter is slower than that of striated muscles.

• Excitability: this is the muscle's natural response to any excitation applied to it.

• Contractility: corresponds to the shortening, thickening and hardening of the muscle. This ability of the muscle is essential for movement.

• Elasticity: refers to the muscle's ability to stretch and return to its initial position when traction ceases.

• Tonicity: also known as muscle tone, this is muscle tension and the slight permanent involuntary contraction in the absence of movement **[14].**

3. Definition of hydatidosis

Hydatidosis or larval echinococcosis is a parasitosis caused by the taenia Echinococcus granulosus sensu lato. The hydatid cyst is the larva (metacestode) that develops in intermediate hosts, in which humans are accidentally included, while the adult form colonises the intestine of the definitive host, mainly the dog **[15].** It is a cosmopolitan disease that affects public health both in terms of frequency and severity. It is particularly prevalent in countries with a rural lifestyle and a tradition of sheep farming **[4].**

4. Pathogenic agent

Echinococcus granulosus sensu lato is the causative agent of hydatid cysts, which are cestodes of the pathelminth family **[2].**

4.1. Taxonomic classification of echinococci

The pathogen belongs to : **[16].**

Kingdom : Animalia

Subdomain: Metazoans

Phylum: Helminthes

Subphylum: Platelminthes

Class: Cestoda

Order : Cyclophyllidea

Family: Taeiinedae

Genus: Echinococcus

Species : granulosus

The taxonomy of Echinococcus (E.) has long been controversial. Based essentially on morphological differences and host-parasite specificity, 16 species and 13 subspecies were initially described. Subsequently, the majority of these taxa were considered to be synonymous with Echinococcus granulosus, and only 4 ratified species should be retained with regard to human and animal pathogenicity: Echinococcus granulosus sensu lato, E. multicularis, E. oligarthus, E. vogeli. Nevertheless, over the last 50 years, significant phenotypic variability has been observed in the field, and at laboratory level, between Echinococcus isolates, particularly those of Echinococcus granulosus, which include differences in: morphology, in vivo and in vitro development, host specificity, pathogenicity, antigenicity, chemical and metabolic composition, proteins and enzymes **[17].**

The application of molecular tools revealed the existence of 10 strains of Echinococcus granulosus. These are Echinococcus granulosus sensu stricto from G1 to G3.

- The G1 strain (dog-sheep): is the most widespread genotype in the world. This strain is commonly found in the liver and lungs, causing echinococcosis in humans, sheep and cattle **[18].**
- G2 strain: Tasmanian sheep strain.
- G3 strain: buffalo strain **[19].**
- The G4 (dog-horse) strain: E. equinus, infects horses, but is not pathogenic in humans.
- The G5 strain (dog-ox): E. ortleppi, this bovine strain rarely infects humans.
- The G6 strain (dog-dromad) **[20].**
- The G7 strain: pig strain.
- The G8 strain: the cervid strain.
- The G9 strain: this genotype has been detected in patients in Poland.
- The G10 strain: a new European genotype **[19].**

3 genotypes of E. granulosus sensu lato, G1 (57.44%), G3 (41.48%) and G6 (1.06%) are responsible for hydatidosis in humans. **[21].**

4.2. Morphology of the parasite

4.2.1. Adult form

The adult Echinococcus granulosus worm is a flatworm measuring between 5 and 8 mm in length. This form is present in the intestine of the definitive host, the dog.

It is made up of :

◊ A cephalic part or scolex: pear-shaped in appearance. It has four rounded suckers, a rostrum and a double crown of hooks. The anterior crown has large hooks, while the posterior crown has small hooks.

The elements of the head allow the worm to attach itself to the intestinal wall of the host.
◊ The body or strobile: made up of three rings or proglottids, the first two of which are immature.

◊ The last ring is a gravid uterus, with unilateral, irregularly alternating genital pores. When mature, it actively detaches from the body with the help of intestinal peristalsis and is then eliminated in the dog's faeces. **[22].**

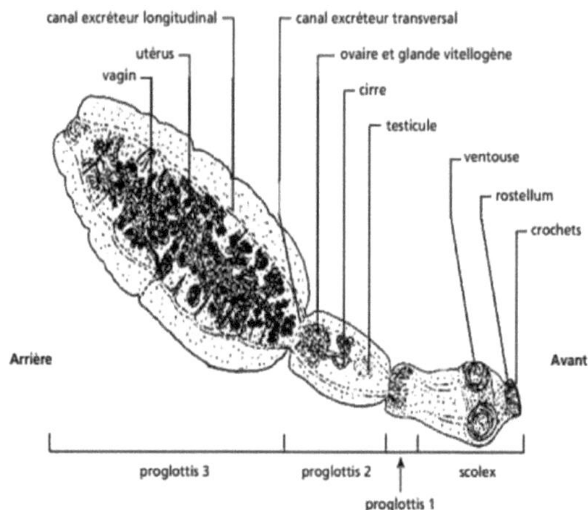

Figure 1: Diagram of the adult form of Echinococcus granulosus **[23].**

4.2.2. Embryophore (egg)

The eggs are ovoid, uncapped and 30 to 40 μm in diameter. They are consisting of a hexacanth embryophore or oncosphere (in the first larval stage), surrounded by a highly resistant keratinised outer envelope, which gives it a dark striated appearance. The outer capsule rapidly disappears once the eggs have been released in the dog's faeces. The survival of the embryophore depends on humidity and temperature conditions. It is highly resistant and can remain infectious for up to a whole year in a damp place at low temperatures (around 4 to 15 degrees Celsius). Echinococcus granulosus eggs are also destroyed by desiccation. At a humidity of 25%, they are destroyed in four days, in one day at 0%, and in less than 5 minutes at 60 - 80 degrees Celsius **[24].**

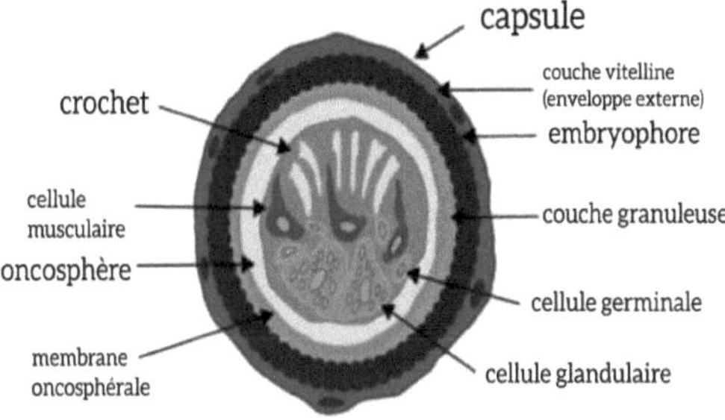

Figure 2. Diagram of an Echinococcus granulosus egg **[25].**

4.2.3. The larval form or hydatid

Also known as the Echinococcus hydatid vesicle. It is an opaque, tense and elastic sphere, varying in diameter up to 30 cm. This cyst is unilocular cavity filled with a liquid under pressure. It is frequently found in the liver and lungs of the intermediate host. However, it can also develop in other organs. locations, such as bones **[26].**

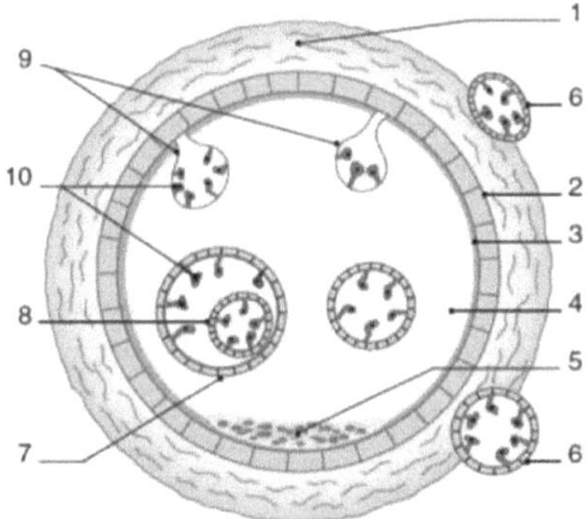

Figure 3: Schematic diagram of the larval form of the hydatid cyst.

1. Reactive adventitia; **2.** cuticle membrane (outer); **3.** proligeral membrane (inner); **4.** Hydatid fluid; **5.** Hydatid sand; **6.** Exogenous daughter vesicle; **7.** Proligeral vesicle (capsule); **8.** Protoscolex; **9.** Endogenous daughter vesicle; **10.**

Little girl's bladder **[27].** The different components of the larval form are presented above.

4.2.3.1. Weed reaction

It is a thick, hard, fibro-conjunctive shell of non-parasitic origin, resulting from the inflammatory reaction of the cells of the parasitised viscera, giving rise to a pericyst. There is a cleavage plane between the adventitia and the hydatid larva **[28].**

4.2.3.2. Double membrane or cystic wall

❖ **The outer membrane or cuticle**

A mucopolysaccharide membrane made up of concentric, stratified and anhistatic chitin lamellae. It is a fragile membrane, with an elasticity that allows it to distend under the pressure exerted by the hydatid fluid. It facilitates the passage of nutrients into the cyst. It also has the function of protecting the parasite from the immune reaction of the intermediate host, the mechanism of which has not yet been elucidated **[22].**

❖ **The germ membrane**

This is a very thin membrane (10 to 15 μm), which lines the inside of the cuticle. It acts as a highly selective filter, allowing antigenic molecules to pass through to the parasitized organism, causing minor anaphylactic reactions such as urticaria.

It plays a number of roles, including the growth of the hydatid, secretion of the hydatid fluid that keeps the hydatid cyst under tension, genesis of the layers of the peripheral cuticle and, in particular, asexual reproduction by polyembryony, by budding from liquid-filled proligeral vesicles (300 to 800 μm), which have no cuticular membrane and remain attached to the proligeral membrane by means of a syncial pedicle. Each vesicle in turn buds, giving rise to around ten protoscolexes measuring 50 to 150 μm, which represent the head of future adult tapeworms.

Endogenous daughter vesicles can rupture and consequently release scolex into the hydatid fluid, as well as detach and remain floating. However, exogenous daughter vesicles derived from fragments of the germ membrane become embedded in the anhistatic cuticle during their formation and vesiculate in turn, giving rise to multiple protoscolexes. This external process is uncommon in humans and can give the hydatid cyst a nippled external appearance **[29].**

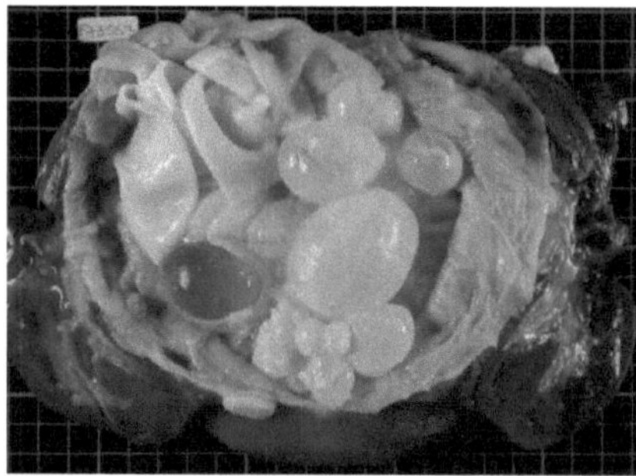

Figure 4. Macroscopic appearance of a renal hydatid cyst with the presence of daughter vesicles **[30].**

4.2.3.3. Hydatid fluid

The lumen of the cyst is filled with a clear, sterile liquid, composed mainly of water (99%), plus a mixture of molecules derived from both the parasite and the host's serum. The hyperpressure inside, which can reach 100 cm of water for a diameter of 10 cm, is a crucial factor in growth and complications such as rupture, which is reduced in old cysts and multivesicular cysts. The liquid represents a favourable culture medium when the hydatid ruptures **[22].**

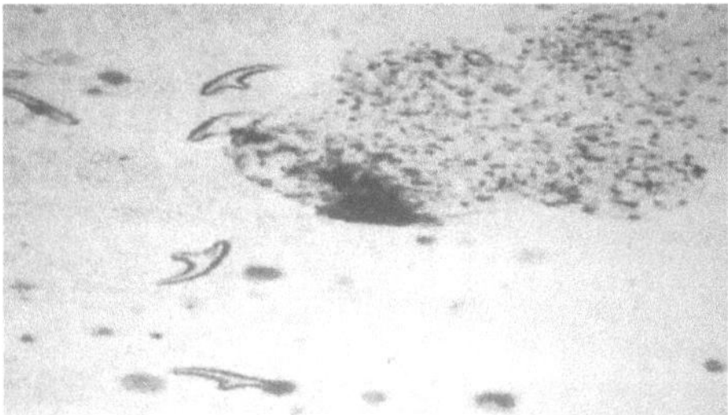

Figure 5. Hydatid fluid with protoscolex and hooks **[31].**

4.2.3.4. Sand hydatique

Hydatid sand is the sloping part of the hydatid, with a sediment composed of elements detached from the germinal membrane: free protoscolexes, ruptured vesicles, dehiscent capsules, daughter vesicles, chitinous hooks emanating from degenerated and destroyed scolexes **[29].**

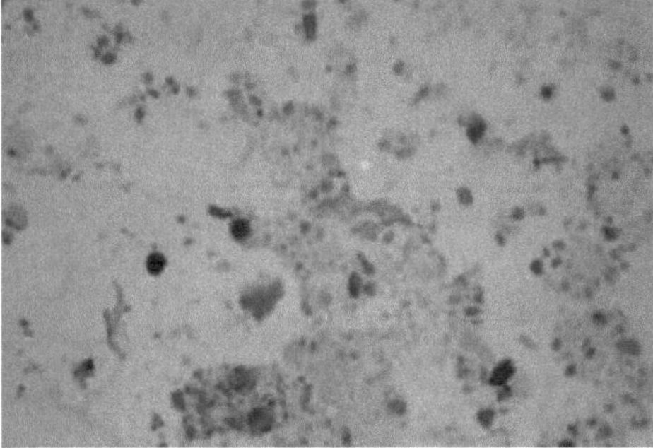

Figure 6. Hydatid sand with hooks **[22].**

5. Geographical breakdown

5.1. In the world

E. granulosus sensu lato is transmitted mainly by dogs and various intermediate hosts. Hydatid cyst is a cosmopolitan disease, present throughout the world except Antarctica, with endemic regions in North Africa, particularly Algeria, Morocco, Libya and Tunisia [32]. In contrast, the highest prevalence in the world, with a rate of 6.6% in men, has been reported in East Africa, in the Turkana outbreak (north-east Kenya) [28].

The Mediterranean basin remains the area where hydatid cysts pose a serious threat, with high prevalence in Spain and certain regions of Italy, Greece and Turkey [32].

A re-emergence of the disease has been observed in several countries in Central Asia, China, Eastern Europe and Israel [33].

South America is an endemic area for cystic echinococcosis (CE), where the disease is widespread in many countries (Peru, Argentina, Bolivia, Uruguay, Chile and the southern part of Brazil) [34].

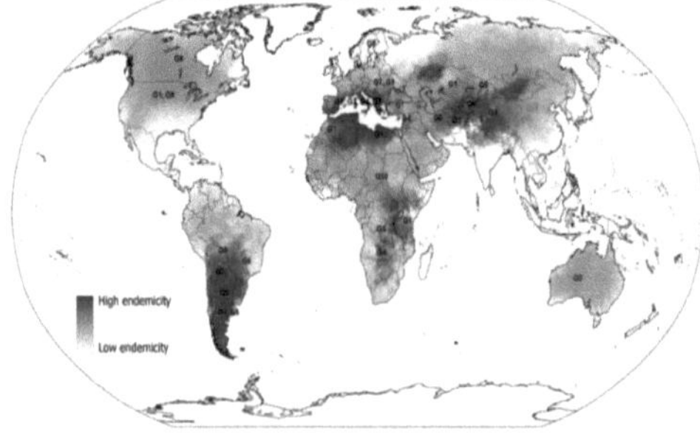

Figure 7. Geographical distribution of cystic echinococcosis worldwide [35].

5.2. At Algeria

In Algeria, EC is a real public health and economic problem. In addition, the disease is transmitted to humans via a sheep/dog cycle [36]. The G1 sheep strain infects sheep, cattle and humans, while the G6 camel strain infects camels. The intermediate hosts represented by farm animals and humans are often infested by dogs, with a prevalence rate of 24.8% for camels, 13.8% for cattle and 6% for horses. The ovine and camelina strains occur in northern and southern Algeria respectively [35]. Research has shown that the prevalence rate of hydatidosis in Algeria is between 3.4 and 4.6 cases per 100,000 inhabitants [37].

6. Cycle

The parasite cycle involves two hosts: a definitive host involving dogs and other canids, and an intermediate host represented by ungulates (sheep, goats, pigs, horses). The definitive hosts become infected by ingesting cyst-bearing viscera. The adult worms reside in the dog's small intestine, which is the main definitive host. They then release eggs which are eliminated into the environment with the dog's excreta [35].The intermediate host becomes infested following ingestion of the eggs, and under the action of enzymes in the stomach and small intestine, the embryophore releases the oncosphere. Bile helps to activate the oncosphere, and it uses its six hooks to pierce the intestinal wall **[24]**. The oncosphere enters the systemic circulation (portal circulation) towards the liver or (in the lymph) towards the lungs, which are the two usual sites for larval development of the parasite **[38]**. Once inside these organs, it loses its hooks and develops into a metacestode or hydatid, generating numerous protoscolexes which, after ingestion, evaginate and attach themselves to the intestinal mucosa of the definitive host, where they develop, becoming adults in 32-80 days, and a new cycle is reproduced **[33]**. Man is an accidental host, providing a biological dead end for the parasite **[24]**.

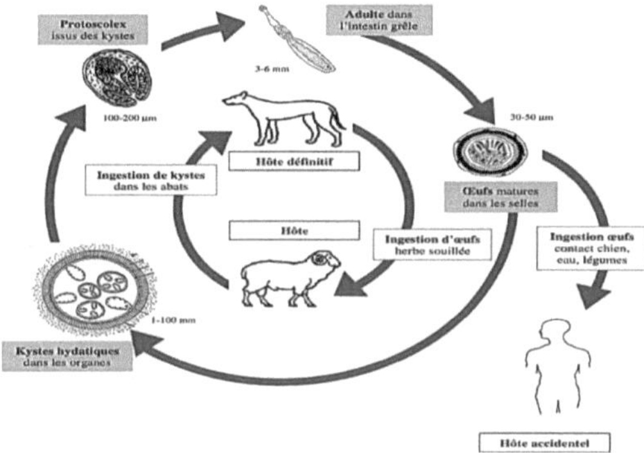

Figure 8. Evolutionary cycle of Echinococcus granulosus **[39]**.

7. Method of contamination

7.1. Mode of contamination of the host definitive

The definitive host (canids and wild carnivores) becomes infected through carnivorism, by ingesting the intermediate host, or the viscera parasitised by fertile hydatids. This is the case in rural areas, where livestock farming is pastoral and herds are heavily parasitised, and where animal viscera from local slaughterhouses serve as a meal for the dogs. This is also the case in sheep pastures, where the corpses of parasitized animals are buried in poorly dug graves, giving dogs access to devour them **[29,40]**.

7.2. Mode of contamination of intermediate hosts

7.2.1. Contamination animal

Domestic herbivores are intermediate hosts, harbouring the larval form of E. granulosus, and are mainly cattle, sheep, goats and camels. These animal species become infected in grasslands by ingesting grass soiled by the faeces of the parasitised definitive host **[41]**.

7.2.2. Human contamination [22,29,40,41,42].

Human infection results from commensalism and cohabitation with the dog population affected by hydatid echinococcosis, particularly in rural areas where there is close contact with dogs. Veterinary surgeons and children are particularly at risk, due to their emotional contact with dogs.Since humans are not prey to canids, they constitute a parasitic dead end. They contract the disease by ingesting the embryonated eggs, in one of two ways:

❖ **Direct route :**

Dogs contaminate humans through licking, or by having their coat stroked when it is soiled with eggs, because when dogs groom themselves, they lick their perianal area, where the eggs accumulate and end up being scattered over their fur with their tongue.

❖ **Indirect route:**

It is spread by ingesting raw plants or water contaminated by the faeces of the definitive host. Eggs are spread passively by wind, rain, rivers, arthropods, human shoes and animal feet.

8. Locations of parasites

Hydatid cysts can develop in any organ. The most common sites are the liver and lungs, but there are also exceptional sites such as the bone, which is rare even in highly endemic areas.

8.1. Predominant locations

8.1.1. Hydatidosis liver

Hepatic hydatidosis is the predominant site of the disease, accounting for two-thirds of cases, and is due to the obligatory portal passage of the larval form of the taenia Echinococcus granulosus. This parasitic disease is very common in North African countries **[43].**

When the embryophore is ingested by the intermediate host, it reaches the mesenteric venous circulation to reach the liver, where it vacuolates and presents a central vesiculation to give a hydatid cyst.

Hepatic echinococcosis is primary and occurs on the right in 65% of cases. It is usually associated with other extrahepatic locations such as the lungs, spleen and peritoneum, in cases where the cyst is multiple **[44].**

8.1.2. Hydatidosis pulmonary

Pulmonary hydatid cysts are caused by the development of hydatids in the lungs, mainly in the right lower lobe **[45].** It is estimated to account for 25 to 40% of human hydatid diseases **[46].**

After ingesting the hexacanth embryos, they find their way into the intestinal lumen, which they then cross to take the chyliferous tract and the portal system. They reach the lungs via the hepatic sinusoids, the inferior vena cava and the right heart chambers **[47].**

The lung is the second most common site after the liver in adults **[48].** However, it is the organ most affected in children, especially as the hepatic filter is porous **[47].**

8.2. Rare locations

8.2.1. Hydatidosis bone

Bone hydatidosis accounts for 0.5 to 2.5% of all cases and is most often found in adults, with a predominance of males. This rarity is justified by the route taken by the hexacanth embryo, which, after digestive absorption, passes through the liver and then the lungs via the haematogenous route, where the capillaries are smaller than the bone capillaries, providing a selective filter. Hydatid cysts in bone are almost always primary, rather than continuous or disseminated. The hard consistency of the bone gives hydatid cysts an anatomical expression that is distinct from that of other localisations. There are no clear boundaries.

The bone location of hydatidosis is predominantly in the spine, which occurs in 44% of cases, but also in the pelvis. In long bones, the hydatid cyst develops in the epiphysis-metaphysis, with secondary extension to the diaphysis, and this can be explained by the parasite's blood tropism **[5,6,8,49].**

8.2.2. Hydatidosis muscle

Muscular localisation is unusual, with an estimated frequency of less than 3%, even in endemic areas.Muscle involvement is most often isolated, and ranks 3rd after liver and lung involvement. It affects the musculature of the chest wall, the pectoralis major muscle, the tailor muscle, the quadriceps and the gluteal muscles **[7,50].**

8.2.3. Hydatidosis cerebral

Hydatidosis develops in the brain in 1 to 2% of cases, and most often affects children (80 to 90% of cases). It may complicate a cardiac location, and among cerebral locations, supratentorial location is thought to be the most frequent **[51,52].**

8.2.4. Hydatidosis

Hydatid cysts of the heart are rare in adults, and even rarer in children. 60% of cardiac hydatid cysts are isolated, and 40% of cases are associated with locations in the liver or lungs. The left ventricle is the most affected since it receives twice as much blood as the right ventricle, usually in the subepicardial layer, and subendocardially in the right heart **[53].**

8.2.5. Hydatidosis renal

Renal localization is rare, even in endemic areas, with an estimated frequency of 5% of visceral forms, although it is the most common localization in the urogenital tract. Hydatid cysts of the kidney are mainly associated with hepatic localisations, and pulmonary localisations in 2 to 5% of cases. It is most often primary and unique, located in the cortex and generally polar. The left kidney is the most commonly affected by hydatidosis **[30].**

8.2.6. Hydatidosis splenic

Hydatid cysts of the spleen rank third, after hydatid cysts of the liver and lungs, as do hydatid cysts of the muscles. Its frequency varies between 2 and 8%. In endemic areas, 50-80% of splenic cystic lesions are of hydatid origin. Splenic contamination occurs in two ways: either via the bloodstream, once the hexacanth embryo has passed through the hepatic and pulmonary filters, or retrograde; from the liver, and via retrograde portal venous circulation, in the case of portal hypertension **[46].**

8.2.7. Hydatidosis pancreatic

This is an exceptional site, and even in highly endemic countries, the incidence is less than 1%. Contamination of the pancreas occurs via the haematogenous route, after passing through the hepatic and pulmonary filters.

Hydatid cysts of the pancreas are isolated in 91% of cases. The location in the gland is usually peripheral (two-thirds of cases). The hydatid is located in the head in 57% of cases, the body in 24% and the tail in 19% **[54].**

8.2.8. Hydatidosis peritoneal

Peritoneal hydatid cysts are rarely primary, due to haematogenous involvement. The form secondary to liver damage is the most common.The frequency of peritoneal location of hydatid cysts varies between 5 and 16% **[55].**

9. Clinical signs

Hydatid echinococcosis is characterised by a slow course and insidious onset.
The appearance of clinical signs depends on :

- ✓ The size of the cyst, however, small cysts <5 cm, well encapsulated and not calcified, remain asymptomatic for several years.
- ✓ The organ affected and the location of the cyst within it.
- ✓ The compressive effect exerted by the cyst on neighbouring structures.
- ✓ The immune status of the intermediate host.
- ✓ Complications secondary to rupture of a primary cyst responsible for dissemination of protoscolex, or induced by superinfection of the cyst **[24].**

9.1. Hydatidosis liver

A hydatid cyst in the liver remains latent for a long time, and is often revealed by pain in the right hypochondrium, a feeling of heaviness, hepatomegaly **[56]** and digestive problems **[38]**. Secondary complications may also arise, such as superinfection leading to the formation of a liver abscess **[57],** which when ruptured in the bile ducts leads to cholangitis, with or without obstructive jaundice, the cyst may also rupture in the lungs, causing pulmonary hydatidosis and bronchial fistula **[56]**, or intraperitoneally (causing secondary hydatidosis), leading to acute peritonitis and anaphylactic shock with a poor prognosis. Compression of the bile ducts and suprahepatic veins can lead to portal hypertension and Budd-Chiari syndrome **[58].**

9.2. Hydatidosis pulmonary

The disease is characterised by a slow, asymptomatic course. The disease is revealed either as a result of general and/or respiratory signs (chest pain, haemoptysis, chronic cough, dyspnoea **[38]**, or when the cyst ruptures, giving rise to febrile episodes, a hacking cough and sputum. However, it is possible for the cyst to become superinfected **[59].**

9.3. Hydatidosis muscle

The clinical form of the condition is represented by a painless, non-inflammatory swelling of the soft tissues, which increases in size over time, without altering the patient's general condition. However, other signs may appear following complications induced by nerve compression, or superinfection of the cyst causing a hot abscess or malignant tumour **[60].**

9.4. Hydatidosis bone

Bone hydatid cysts evolve slowly **[33]**. The clinical picture is not very suggestive, depending on the location of the cyst, and may present as pain and swelling **[61].**

The onset of the disease may be attributed to superinfection of the cyst, or to the compressive effect of the cyst, leading to neurovascular lesions **[33].**

A cyst located in the long bones can lead to fracture **[28]**, which in turn can reveal its presence **[33].**Spinal deformity, soft tissue swelling, pathological fractures and paraplegia are the tell-tale signs of vertebral hydatidosis, which has a dreadful prognosis **[28].**

Discreet limping on walking is observed when the cyst is located in the lower limbs or pelvis **[61].**

9.5. Hydatidosis pancreatic

The clinical picture depends on the location of the cyst, with retentional jaundice and a palpable epigastric abdominal mass, but abdominal pain above the umbilical region seems to be the main reason for consultation. Complications include cyst suppuration, haemorrhagic episodes and allergic reactions resulting from intra- or retroperitoneal rupture **[54].**

9.6. Hydatidosis splenic

The disease progresses slowly and remains asymptomatic for several years. The clinical form often encountered is splenomegaly and pain in the left hypochondrium **[62].**

The cyst may be complicated by abscessation or rupture in the pleura, stomach or colon **[63].**

9.7. Hydatidosis cerebral

The clinical picture is one of headaches, dizziness and altered consciousness. Depending on the location of the cyst, specific neurological deficits may be associated with it

[38].

9.8. Hydatidosis

Heart rhythm disorders, palpitations, exertional dyspnoea, angina and haemoptysis are the most common clinical signs.Possible complications include systemic and pulmonary embolisms, myocardial tears and conduction disorders **[64].**

9.9. Hydatidosis renal

Clinically, it is manifested by a pain syndrome and a tumour syndrome. Hydaturia seems to be a specific sign of renal hydatid cysts, which is related to the retroperitoneal development of the cyst, testifying to the rupture of the cyst in the excretory tract **[65].**

9.10. Hydatidosis peritoneal

Abrupt rupture of the cyst may be manifested by ascites or an acute abdominal syndrome, but the clinical picture is still dominated by pain in the situs, which may be associated with vomiting, and may even lead to deterioration in the patient's general condition. Retentional jaundice due to compression of the bile ducts or bilio-cystic fistula may be encountered **[55].**

10. Diagnosis

10.1. Diagnosis

10.1.1. Non specific biological signs

Hydatidosis is a helminthiasis with a life cycle requiring intra-tissue passage, which can induce blood hypereosinophilia, which is a biological sign defined as greater than 500 eosinophilic polynuclear cells/mm^3 . However, this level varies according to the stage of infestation, increasing as the body responds to antigenic stimulation. It reaches a maximum in a few weeks to a few months during tissue passage, then decreases **[66].**

Neutrophil hyperleukocytosis indicates superinfection of the hydatid cyst **[45].**

10.1.2. Parasitological diagnosis direct

The direct search for the parasite in bronchial fluids after vomiting, or in pleural fluid, or any other sample containing protoscolex and hydatid hooks, constitutes the diagnosis of certainty. However, it is rarely carried out in everyday practice, and is only occasionally requested. Apart from diagnostic purposes, this research allows us to study the viability of protoscolex and the fertility of cysts. This fertility is generally implicated in the appearance of possible secondary hydatidosis, which arises as a result of spontaneous or accidental rupture, after a traumatic or post-therapeutic procedure, and consequently the release of viable protoscolex, which join other organs **[67].**

10.1.3. Immunological diagnosis indirect

Hydatid serology is based on the detection of specific anti-parasitic antibodies in the blood. It is an essential step in diagnosis, and in particular in the detection of hydatid recurrences, through the presence of G4 immunoglobulins, which are thought to be markers of hydatid recurrence, whereas G2 immunoglobulins are linked to primary infections. It is used to guide the diagnosis of echinococcosis using the following methods:

❖ **Immunoelectrophoresis**

This method is less and less used because of its cumbersome nature, but it is highly specific. It highlights arc 5.

❖ **Enzyme-Linked Immunosorbent Assay (ELISA)**

The sensitivity of enzyme immunoassay makes it the complementary method of choice, in addition to immunoelectrophoresis.

❖ **Indirect haemagglutination, electrosynthesis,immunofluorescence and western blot**

These are also high-performance techniques that are commonly used **[1].** It is important to combine two techniques: one quantitative (ELISA) and the other qualitative (Western Blot). The diagnosis is confirmed when both techniques are positive with a significant rate. Hydatid serology is used to determine whether a hydatid cyst is viable or inactive.**[68].**

10.2. Medical imaging

10.2.1. Radiography

Standard X-rays can rule out bone involvement **[69].** However, a definite diagnosis can only be made by histological study of the lesion, because it is difficult to confirm the diagnosis of echinococcosis on a bone lesion revealed by X-ray and clarified by CT scan **[5].**

Radiography most often shows poorly limited lytic areolar images, giving the classic honeycomb appearance, and calcifications in the case of an aged hydatid cyst **[8,69].**It should be noted that in most cases, a positive diagnosis of pulmonary hydatid cyst can be made using a chest X-ray **[47].**

10.2.2. Ultrasound

This is the examination of choice for diagnosing hydatid cysts. It indicates the fluid nature of the swelling and its location. It is used to diagnose echinococcosis in typical cases. Hypoechogenic pseudo-tissue images correspond to hydatid sludge **[69]**.Abdominal ultrasound and thoracoabdominal ultrasound play an important role in the positive diagnosis of hydatid cysts in the liver and then the lungs **[47,58]**.The two classifications of hydatidosis are those of Gharbi **(Table I)** and the World Health Organisation (WHO) **[70]**. According to Gharbi's classification, there are five sonographic aspects of the hydatid cyst as shown in the following table:

Types	Ultrasound aspects
Type I	A liquid mass with a clean wall.
Type II	Membrane detachment.
Type III	Multivesicular.
Type IV	Pseudotumoral lesion.
Type V	Hydatid cyst with calcified wall.

Table I: Gharbi classification **[71]**.

In 2002, a classification was suggested by the WHO, with the aim of better selecting patients for percutaneous treatment. This classification uses the fertile or non-fertile character of the hydatid cyst of the liver, and its transitional character:

• group 1 (infertile cystic lesion).

• group 2 (fertile hydatid cysts): type cystic echinococcosis 1 and type cystic echinococcosis 2.

• group 3 (transitional lesion): type cystic echinococcosis 3.

• group 4 (inactive lesion): type cystic echinococcosis 4 and type cystic echinococcosis 5 **[70]**.

10.2.3. Computed tomography (CT)

CT can be used to make a positive diagnosis of cerebral hydatid cysts **[51]**. It is an examination that can be used to determine the hydatid nature of a mass, in the case of ultrasound type IV. It is also useful for studying the relationship with neighbouring organs, vessels and the urinary tract **[72]**. The constraint faced by CT is the same as that faced by ultrasound, because there are atypical forms, where the mass is not clearly liquid, which hinders the obvious identification of a vesicle and/or membrane structure **[69]**.

10.2.4. Magnetic resonance imaging (MRI)

MRI is the imaging technique of choice for soft tissue hydatid pathology **[15]**. It is also used for bone hydatid cysts **[49]**, but is usually reserved for cases where the diagnosis remains doubtful. It allows the location of the lesion and its adjacent relationships to be determined. It can also reveal any vertebral involvement associated with a lesion of the urinary tract **[72]**.

11. Treatment

11.1. Treatment surgical

Surgery plays a vital role in the management of this parasitosis, as it alone can lead to a cure **[24]**.This therapeutic modality aims to :

✓ Inactivate the infectious compartment of the parasite, including the scolex, and the germinal membrane.

✓ Reduce the frequency of parasite dissemination.
✓ Manage the residual cavity.

Surgical interventions are either radical or conservative approaches; the radical approach aims to remove the entire cyst, including the peri-cyst, making the technique more reliable, with less risk of recurrence, but with a significant incidence of post-operative complications, whereas the conservative approach aims to extract only the contents of the parasitic cyst, while preserving the peri-cyst, the latter being safe prior to surgery, but with a significant rate of recurrence. Treatment of the residual cavity involves lining, marsupialization and omentoplasty **[73]**.Patients who can undergo surgery are those who have :
✓ A secondary complication of bacterial superinfection of the cyst, or compression of neighbouring structures induced by the cyst, or following a possible communication with the bile ducts.

✓ Large hepatic cysts with multiple daughter cysts, by partial hepatectomy, pericystectomy, open cystectomy with or without omnetoplasty.

✓ Lung cysts by lobectomy, extrusion of cysts using the barrette technique, pericystectomy **[24]**.

✓ Muscle cysts (pericystectomy) **[60]**.

✓ Bone cysts (carcinological excision of hydatid lesions) **[61]**.
✓ Cysts in the spleen (total splenectomy is the preferred technique, although partial splenectomy and enucleation with omnetoplasty are not excluded from the choice) **[46]**.

✓ Peritoneal cysts, where surgery aims to treat cysts in the peritoneum and primary cysts simultaneously **[74]**.

✓ Pancreatic cysts: treatment remains primarily surgical, with the choice of technique depending on the location of the cyst and whether or not there is a cysto-ductal fistula **[54]**.

✓ Cardiac hydatidosis: curable by cystectomy, pericystectomy, followed by lining of the residual cavity **[75]**.

✓ Renal hydatidosis: partial pericystectomy or resection of the protruding dome, offering surgeons the techniques of choice, and which make it possible to obtain satisfactory results without damaging the renal parenchyma **[65]**.

✓ Cerebral hydatidosis: neurosurgical treatment **[76].**

However, surgery remains limited and is contraindicated during pregnancy and in patients with diseases (cardiac, renal, hepatic, etc.), as well as in patients with cysts that are small, difficult to access, non-viable or calcified.

11.2. Treatment medical

Medical management is a non-invasive treatment option that can be used for patients of any age, although it is more effective in younger than in older patients. It appears to be more effective on small, thin-walled cysts that are not superinfected or complicated by secondary involvement. On the other hand, daughter cysts, contained in mother cysts, appear to be less sensitive to this treatment **[24].**

Patients presenting a contraindication to surgery, or with multiple cysts that are difficult to access, or an inoperable form of hydatidosis of hepatic, pulmonary, peritoneal or cerebral origin, may be eligible for medical treatment.At the same time, this treatment modality offers an alternative in highly endemic areas where access to other treatment options is limited by the lack of healthcare facilities.In addition, it has been shown that in patients undergoing surgery, prior administration of Benzimidazole derivatives will soften the cysts by reducing intra-cystic pressure, thereby facilitating the procedure and removal of the cysts. Secondly, this treatment reduces the viability of protoscolex and cysts, helping to prevent recurrence. Chemotherapy using Benzimidazole derivatives (Albendazole, Mebendazole) acts by altering the germ layer of the parasite, depriving it of glucose and causing cellular autolysis **[77].**

The prescribed dosage is :

- Albendazole: 10mg/kg administered orally, twice daily, for 3 to 6 months, at 14-day intervals.
- Mebendazole: 40mg/kg to 50mg/kg administered orally, three times a day, for three to six months **[24].**

According to pharmacokinetic data, concomitant administration of the drug with a high-fat meal will result in better bioavailability of the compound.

Chemotherapy should not be given to pregnant women because of its teratogenic effect, particularly during the first trimester, or to patients who have undergone chemotherapy. liver or bone marrow failure, or with large cysts prone to rupture, or inactive or calcified cysts **[77]**.

11.3. Percutaneous treatment (puncture, aspiration, injection, reaspiration)

Percutaneous treatment guided by imaging, particularly ultrasound, was introduced in the mid-1980s **[24].** The technique is performed in three stages: After establishing strict asepsis rules appropriate to the procedure, and under locoregional anaesthesia, the technique is performed as follows: Initially, using a fine needle and under ultrasound control, the cyst is punctured to aspirate the fluid it contains. This allows the diagnosis of hydatidosis to be confirmed, by highlighting the mobile protoscolex, and also to look for the presence of any fistulas.Once the cyst contents have been extracted, a scolicidal agent (20-30% hypertonic saline or 95% alcohol) is injected.After 20 to 30 minutes, the bark-killing solution is aspirated again **[60]**.This less traumatic technique would be offered to all patients with inoperable cysts, or for whom surgery is contraindicated. The locations concerned by this therapeutic option are as follows: hepatic, splenic, renal, bony or peritoneal.If relapses occur after surgery or medical treatment, puncture-aspiration-injection-reaspiration (PAIR) could be considered as an alternative treatment. Pregnant women with a symptomatic form of hydatidosis could also benefit from PAIR, but given the coverage by chemotherapy involving Albendazole, the technique seems to be restricted in this case.Echoguided PAIR is combined with Benzimidazole derivatives to reduce complications caused by secondary echinococcosis. The recommended molecules are Albendazole and Mebendazole administered 4 days before the procedure, for 1 and 3 months respectively. Treatment by PAIR is still contraindicated in cases of pulmonary hydatidosis, hepatic cysts that are difficult to access or superficial, due to the risk of dissemination of the parasite contents into the abdominal cavity, and in cases of cysts with multiple septal divisions (honeycomb cysts), calcified cysts, or cysts communicating with the biliary tree [24].

12. Prophylaxis

Interrupting the natural life cycle of Echincoccus granulsus is inconceivable without implementing prophylactic measures appropriate to the local or regional context concerned **[1]**.

12.1. Permanent host (dog)

Dogs become infected by eating the parasitised viscera of herbivores. It is therefore essential to incinerate offal carrying hydatids **[22]**. The measures adopted to eradicate this disease can be summed up as the culling of stray dogs and the treatment of domestic dogs with Praziquantel **[62]**.

12.2. Intermediate host (sheep)

Veterinary control of cattle slaughter is an essential prophylactic measure in the fight against hydatidosis **[22]**.Vaccination of domestic intermediate hosts with a recombinant Echinococcus granulosus antigen (the EG95 vaccine) offers encouraging prospects for controlling this parasite. However, its cost remains a problem, particularly as this parasitic disease is rife in rural areas where the population is of low socio-economic status **[78]**.

12.3. Accidental host (human)

Individual prevention consists of limiting promiscuity between humans and dogs, especially children, who are particularly exposed through emotional contact (petting and licking by the dog). It is therefore essential to wash hands thoroughly after any contact with the definitive host.Human contact with the taenia Echinococcus granulosus can be indirect through the ingestion of fruit and vegetables soiled by dog faeces, so it is essential to carefully wash plants intended to be eaten raw, such as strawberries and radishes **[29]**.

PART II
PRACTICAL

CHAPTER II
MATERIALS AND METHODS

1. Type and scope of the study

This is a retrospective and descriptive study of 5 cases of osteomuscular hydatid cysts, collected in the orthopaedics and traumatology department of the Benflis Touhami university hospital in Batna, over a period of 10 years, from January 2012 to December 2022.

2. Aims of the study

The main aim of this study is to fill the gap in data on the epidemiological profile of osteo-muscular hydatidosis in the Batna region. The secondary aim of our work is to highlight the risk and prognostic factors for hydatid cysts of bone and muscle.

3. Study population

3.1. Inclusion criteria

The patients recruited in this study are those with an osteo-muscular hydatid cyst, confirmed and explored by medical imaging, whose records are complete and documented.

3.2. Exclusion criteria

✓ Files that could not be used, including 4 patients with osteo-muscular hydatidosis, were eliminated.

✓ Diagnosis mentioned outside the study period.

✓ Patients with a hydatid cyst located outside the bone or muscle.

4. Data collection

The files of patients with osteomuscular hydatidosis were processed on the basis of a pre-established information sheet containing epidemiological, clinical, radiological, biological and therapeutic variables.

5. Data analysis

The data collected was entered and analysed using SPSS 2021 software. We propose to carry out a comparative study between the results we obtained and other research work similar to ours.

6. Ethical considerations

Free and informed consent was obtained from each patient, professional secrecy was safeguarded, and confidentiality and anonymity were de rigueur.

7. Comments

Comment N°1 :

The patient was 30 years old and from Batna. Her surgical history included a cholecystectomy 4 years ago and 5 caesarean sections, the last of which was 3 months ago. She was admitted to the orthopaedics and traumatology department for surgical treatment of a hydatid cyst in the right thigh.

❖ **Clinical examination :**

On general examination, the patient was conscious, haemodynamically and respiratory stable, apyretic, with good hydration and good skin and mucous membrane colouration.

❖ **Biological check-up :**

- Haemogram: eosinophil count was normal.
- C-reactive protein (CRP) was negative.
- Hydatid serology showed progressive hydatidosis.

❖ **Radiological examination :**

- Ultrasound of the thigh revealed a suspected abscess.
- MRI of the right thigh showed a cystic-like image suggestive of a hydatid cyst of the right vastus medialis muscle, type II according to Gharbi's classification **(Figure 9).**

- Angioscan of the lower limbs showed :

✓ An intramuscular cystic formation of the right vastus medialis muscle, in the lower third, with a thin wall, fluid content, and well-limited detachment of the proligeral membrane.

✓ Permeable vascular axis **(figure 10).**

- The chest X-ray was unremarkable **(Figure 11).**

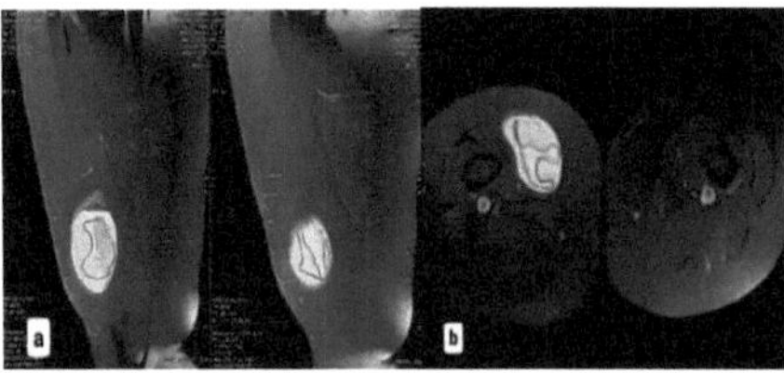

Figure 9 (a,b). MRI of the right thigh showing a hydatid cyst of the right vastus medialis muscle.

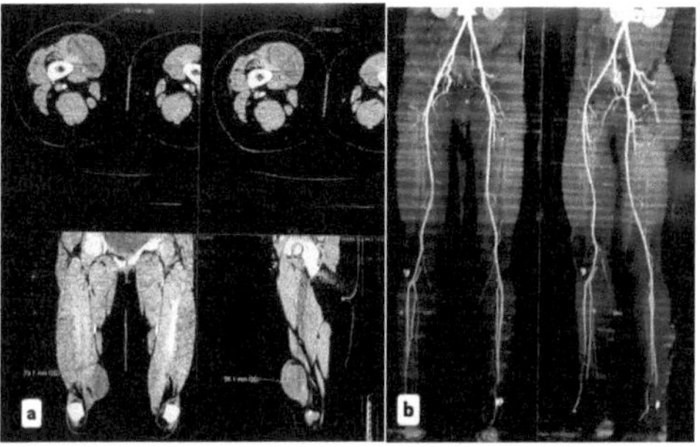

Figure 10 (a,b). Angioscan of the lower limbs.

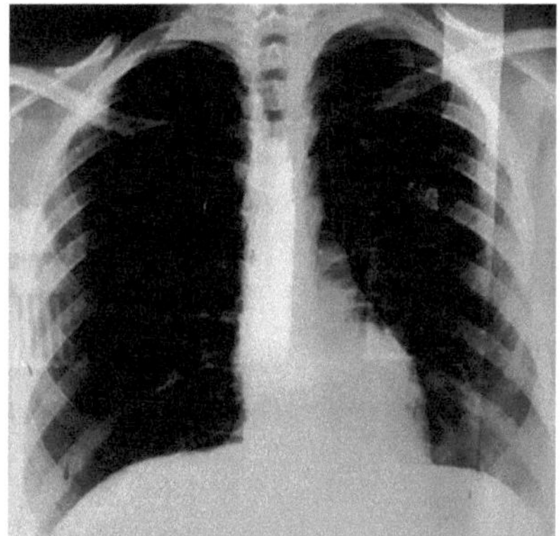

Figure 11. Normal chest X-ray.

❖ **Drug treatment :**

The patient did not receive any anti-helminthic treatment.

❖ **Surgical treatment :**

- The patient underwent surgical removal of the hydatid cyst.

- Investigation revealed a cystic mass in the vastus medialis muscle.

Comment N°2 :

The patient is 38 years old and from Batna. He had undergone surgery in 2011 and 2015 for a hydatid cyst in the sacral region and the root of the right lower limb. He was admitted to the orthopaedics and traumatology department for a recurrence of a hydatid cyst in the right sacroiliac region and the root of the right lower limb.

❖ **Clinical examination :**

- General examination revealed a healthy, haemodynamically stable patient with good mucocutaneous colouration.

- The locomotor examination revealed two clean, good-quality operation scars. One was on the root of the right lower limb, and the other on the right paraspinal lumbar region.

Palpation revealed a palpable, painless mass in the root of the right lower limb, roughly rounded, about 6 cm in diameter, soft and mobile in relation to the superficial and deep layers. The limb was warm and well coloured.

The rest of the examination was unremarkable.

❖ **Biological check-up :**

- The blood count showed no hypereosinophilia.
- Hydatid serology was negative.

❖ **Radiological examination :**

- The ultrasound revealed :

✓ Fluid collection at the surgical sites (the sacral region and the root of the right lower limb).

✓ An intramuscular fluid collection in the right buttock, suggestive of a probable hydatid cyst.

- The abdomino-pelvic CT scan showed: **(Figure 12)**

✓ Poorly limited right iliac osteolysis, with involvement of the right sacroiliac joint and pre-sacral extension.

✓ A round multicompartmental cystic lesion in the gluteal region and the root of the right thigh, suggestive of a recurrence of the hydatid cyst.

✓ Fluid collections at the surgical sites.

- X-rays of the pelvis showed a multilocular osteolytic lesion of the upper end of the left femur **(Figure 13).**

- The chest X-ray showed no other location **(Figure 14).**

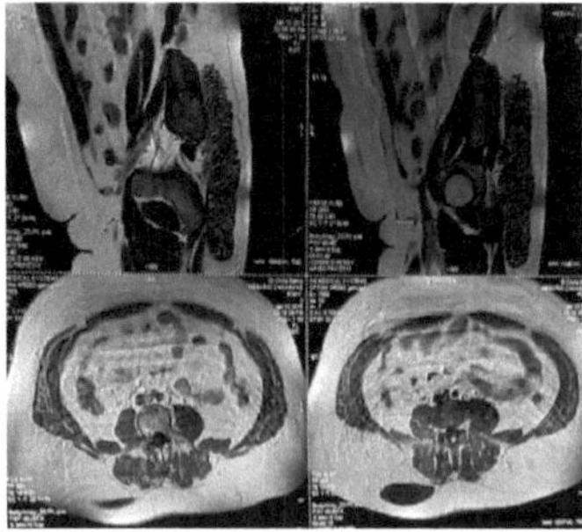

Figure 12. Abdominal and pelvic CT scan.

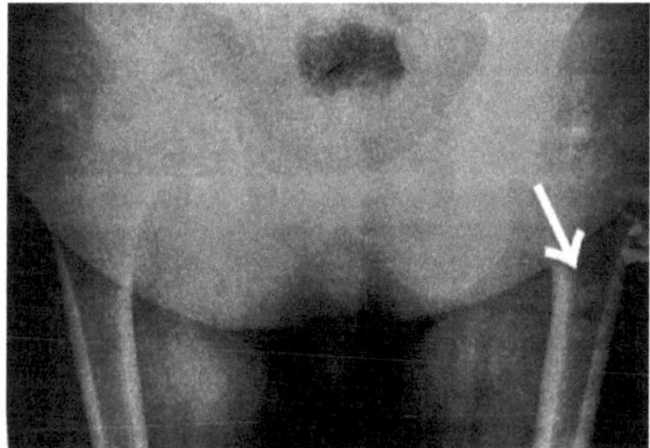

Figure 13. Radiograph of the pelvis showing a multilocular osteolytic lesion.

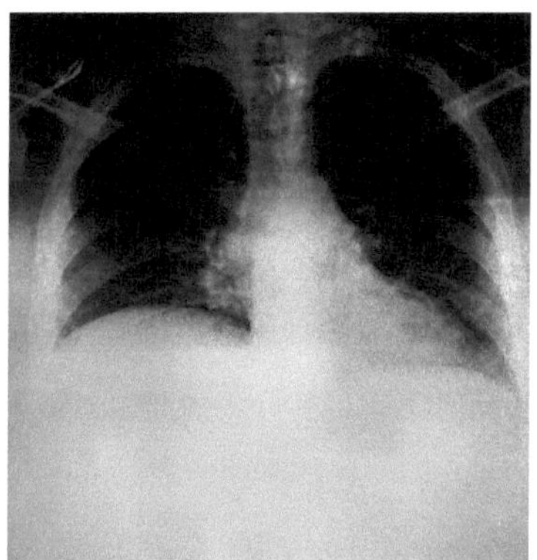

Figure 14. Chest X-ray with no abnormalities.

❖ **Drug treatment :**

The patient was not treated with nematocides.

❖ **Surgical treatment :**

✓ Surgical report :

The procedure was as follows:

- Skin incision under the skin.
- 1er time: right sacroiliac region.
- Puncture and aspiration of hydatid fluid.
- Wash thoroughly with hydrogen peroxide.
- Flat-by-flat closure on suction Redon drain.
- 2nd stage: right inguinal region.
- Skin incision under the skin.
- Aspiration of hydatid fluid.

- Wash thoroughly with hydrogen peroxide.
- Close plane by plane.

Comment N°3 :

The patient was a 36-year-old from Batna. He was admitted to the trauma department for treatment of a recurrent hydatid cyst on the medial side of the left thigh.

❖ **History:**

- The patient had no notable medical history.

- He has been operated on 3 times for a hydatid cyst on the inside of his left thigh, most recently a year ago.

❖ **Clinical examination :**

- On general examination, the patient was conscious, apyretic, haemodynamically stable and in good general condition.

- Locomotor examination revealed a surgical scar on the medial aspect of the left thigh.

- The patient had no pain on palpation and no signs of inflammation in the left thigh.

- Muscular examination showed that the popliteal and pedal pulses were perceptible bilaterally and symmetrically.

- The neurological examination was unremarkable.

❖ **Biological check-up :**

- The blood count was normal.
- The leucocyte count was 8,000 cells/m^3.
- Hydatid serology was positive.

❖ **Radiological examination :**

- MRI of the left thigh showed intra- and inter-muscular hydatid cysts in the medial compartment.

- The chest X-ray was without abnormality **(Figure 15).**

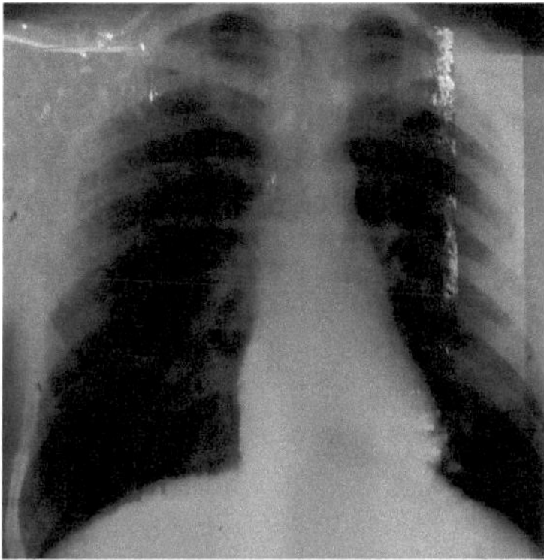

Figure 15. Chest X-ray to rule out a pulmonary location.

❖ **Treatment :**

The patient was treated surgically, without the need for antihelminthic therapy (in particular Benzimidazole derivatives).

✓ Surgical report :

- Under spinal anaesthetic and supine position.
- The operation consisted of an iterative incision.
- Dissection along the path of the cysts, which are located in the adductor magnus muscle.
- Removal of the three cysts, with copious washing with isotonic saline.
- Close plane by plane.
- Aseptic dressing.
- Surgical specimens were sent for anatomopathological examination.

Comment N° 4 :

A 51-year-old woman from Khenchela was admitted to the traumatology department for treatment of a recurrent hydatid cyst in the root of the right thigh.

❖ **History:**
- No particular medical history.
- Operated on 3 years ago for a hydatid cyst in the root of the right thigh.

❖ **History of the disease :**

It dates back three months to the recurrence of a hydatid cyst, with the appearance of a firm, mobile swelling that gradually increased in size.

❖ **Clinical examination :**

-The patient was conscious, cooperative, haemodynamically stable and in good general condition.

-The examination also revealed a firm, mobile mass measuring 4cm, without pain or signs of inflammation on the inner side of the right thigh.

-Motor skills and sensation in the lower limbs were unremarkable.

❖ **Biological check-up :**

- The blood count showed a normal white blood cell count.

- Hydatid serology was negative.

❖ **Radiological examination :**

showed two superficial cystic lesions, subfascial, in the root of the right thigh.

❖ **Treatment :**

The patient had undergone surgery, but had not received any antihelminthic treatment (in particular Benzimidazole derivatives).

Comment N°5 :

He is a 24-year-old man from Batna. He was admitted to the trauma department with pain on the outside of his right thigh. He was diagnosed with osteomuscular hydatidosis of the pelvis and right thigh.

❖ **Background:**

- He had no particular medical history.

- Operated on a year ago for a hydatid cyst in the right thigh.

❖ **Clinical examination :**

- On clinical examination, the patient was conscious, apyretic, cooperative, haemodynamically stable and in good general condition.

- Examination of the cephalic and thoracoabdominal extremities was unremarkable.

- Examination of the musculoskeletal system was normal.

❖ **Biological check-up :**

- The blood count was unremarkable.

- Leukocytes were 7400 elements/m^3.

- Hydatid serology was negative.

❖ **Radiological examination :**

- X-rays of the pelvis showed osteo-muscular hydatidosis of the right hemi pelvis, extending to the thigh root muscle via fistulous tracts **(Figure 16).**

- The chest X-ray was normal **(Figure 17).**

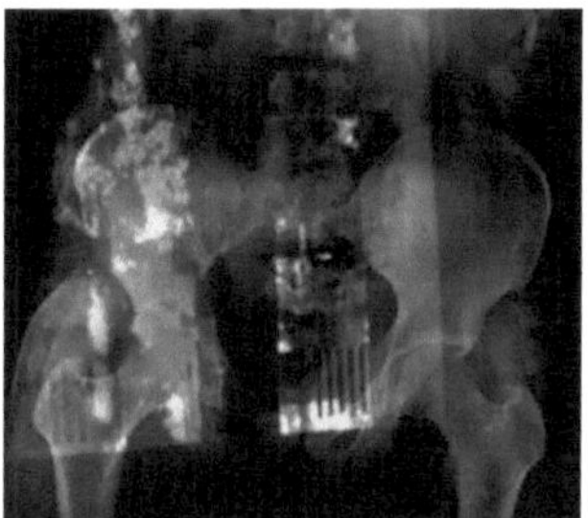

Figure 16. Radiograph of the pelvis showing osteomuscular hydatidosis.

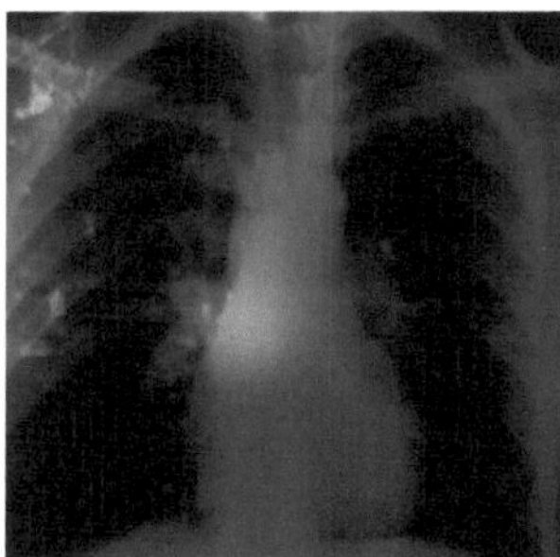

Figure 17. Chest X-ray with no abnormalities.

❖ **Treatment:**

The patient had undergone surgery, but had not received antihelminthic treatment (in particular Benzimidazole derivatives).

CHAPTER III
RESULTS

During our retrospective study, from 2012 to 2022, in the orthopaedic surgery department of the Benflis Touhami university hospital in Batna, five files were studied in order to carry out this work and gather as much information as possible on hydatid disease affecting bone and muscle **(see Table II).**

1. Epidemiological study

1.1. Age

The average age of our patients was 35.80 years, ranging from 24 to 51 years.

1.2. Sex

The distribution of hydatidosis cases by sex is illustrated in Figure 18 below:

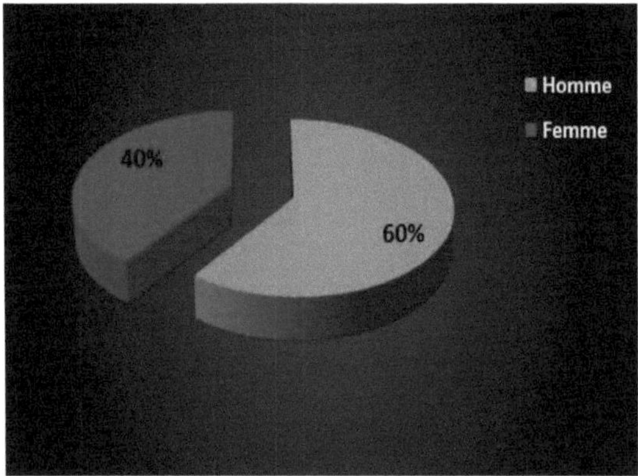

Figure 18. Breakdown of patients by sex.

The distribution of the disease according to sex in Figure 18 shows a clear male predominance, with a percentage of 60% compared with 40% for women.

1.3. Geographical origin

The results relating to the distribution of hydatidosis cases according to geographical origin are illustrated in Figure 19 below:

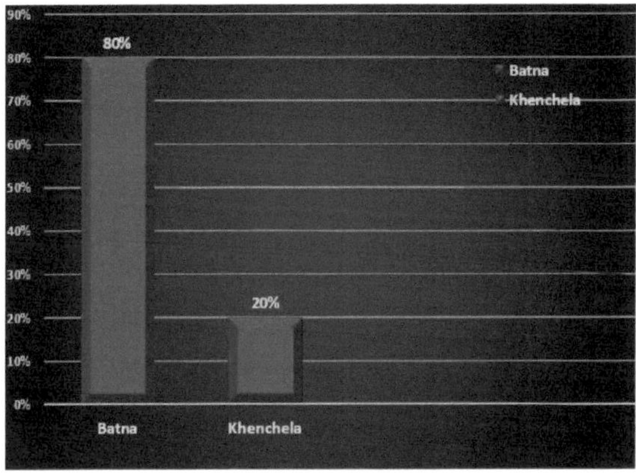

Figure 19. Distribution of hydatidosis cases by geographical origin.

All our patients are 80% from Batna, and only one from Khenchela (20%).

1.4. Location

The percentages of hydatid cyst locations found in our study are shown in Figure 20 below:

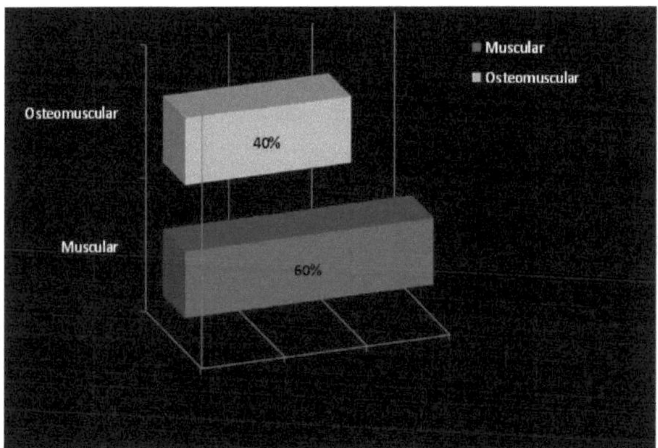

Figure 20: Distribution of hydatidosis cases by organ affected.

In our study, 60% of patients presented with a primary muscular hydatid cyst, compared with 40% with concomitant osteo-muscular involvement. Nevertheless, we
We did not record any cases of primary bone hydatidosis.

1.5. Recidivism

Data on recidivism are shown in Figure 21 below:

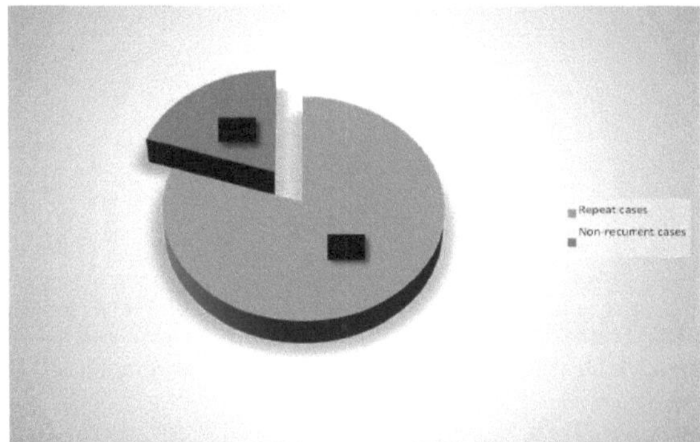

Figure 21. Distribution of hydatidosis cases according to recurrence.

Figure 21 shows that the percentage of recurrent cases is higher than the percentage of non-recurrent cases, i.e. 80% compared with 20%.

1.6. Antecedents

Most of our patients had no particular medical history, while 80% had a surgical history of recurrent hydatid cysts.

2. Clinical examination

2.1. General signs

All the patients in our series were healthy, haemodynamically stable, apyretic and had good mucocutaneous colouration.

2.2. Examination of the musculoskeletal system

Examination of the musculoskeletal system revealed the absence of inflammatory signs in all our patients. This examination was normal in 2 patients, but there were particularities in the other 3, for example:

- Case 2:

- A palpable, painless, roughly rounded mass, about 6 cm in diameter, with a soft, mobile consistency.

- The member was warm and colourful.
- Two scars from surgical removal of two hydatid cysts.

▪ Case 3:
- Presence of a scar from surgery to remove a hydatid cyst.
▪ Case 4:
- Firm, mobile, painless mass measuring 4 cm.

The neurological examination was unremarkable in all patients.

3. Paraclinical examination

3.1. Biology

❖ **Orientation exams :**

- The blood count showed no hypereosinophilia.

- CRP was negative in patients who underwent an inflammatory work-up.

❖ **Direct parasitological examination :**

Scolex was not detected on the surgical specimens of any of the patients in our series.

❖ **Indirect immunological examination :**

- Hydatid serology came back positive in 2 out of 5 patients, in one of whom the immunological diagnosis showed progressive hydatidosis.

- In the case of the other 3 patients, the results came back negative.

3.2. Radiology

❖ **Standard radiography :**

Standard radiography was performed in 3 of our patients. Case 2 showed a multilocular osteolytic lesion. In case 4, it showed two cystic lesions in the root of the right thigh, suggestive of muscular hydatidosis. Case 5 showed osteomuscular hydatidosis.

❖ **Ultrasound :**

Ultrasound examination of the thigh revealed a suspicion of muscle abscess in case 1, but revealed osteo-muscular fluid collections in case 2.

❖ **MRI :**

MRI of the thigh was performed in only 2 patients. It showed an image with a cystic appearance suggestive of a muscular hydatid cyst.

❖ **CT :**

CT scans were performed in cases 1 and 2, to identify the location of cystic muscle lesions, osteolytic lesions and fluid collections.

❖ **Chest X-ray :**

All our patients returned without any particularities, thus ruling out another location for the hydatid cyst.

4. Treatment :

In our series, not all patients received antihelminthic treatment. However, they all underwent surgery.

Table II. Epidemiological, clinical, biological, radiological and therapeutic characteristics of the 5 patients followed for osteomuscular hydatidosis.

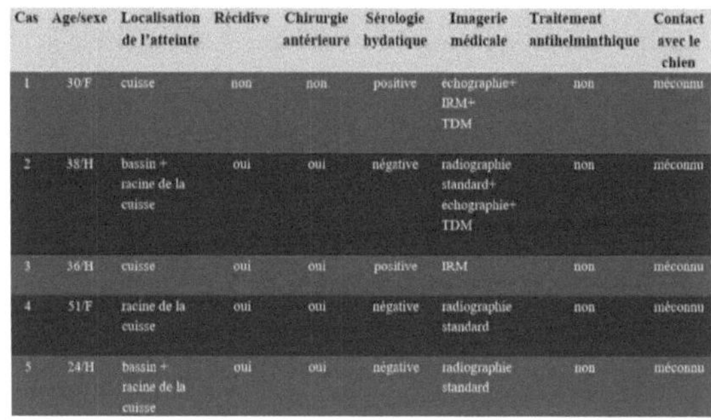

Cas	Age/sexe	Localisation de l'atteinte	Récidive	Chirurgie antérieure	Sérologie hydatique	Imagerie médicale	Traitement antihelminthique	Contact avec le chien
1	30/F	cuisse	non	non	positive	échographie+ IRM+ TDM	non	méconnu
2	38/H	bassin + racine de la cuisse	oui	oui	négative	radiographie standard+ échographie+ TDM	non	méconnu
3	36/H	cuisse	oui	oui	positive	IRM	non	méconnu
4	51/F	racine de la cuisse	oui	oui	négative	radiographie standard	non	méconnu
5	24/H	bassin + racine de la cuisse	oui	oui	négative	radiographie standard	non	méconnu

CHAPTER IV
DISCUSSION

Hydatidosis, also known as hydatid disease, is a parasitic disease caused by the larval stage of the Echinococcus granulosus parasite. It occurs mainly in regions where sheep farming is common. Hydatid cysts can be found in various tissues of the human body, mainly in the liver and lungs, but rarely in other organs **[79]**. The main risk factors are poor hygiene and direct contact with dogs **[8]**. It is a highly endemic disease in North African countries, including Algeria, particularly in rural areas where there is a high risk of transmission of infection **[80]**. The muscular hydatid cyst is a rare site **[60]**, representing less than 3% of all hydatidoses **[69]**. According to several authors, it ranks 3ème after the liver and lungs **[50]**. This rarity is explained by the parasitic cycle of the Echinococcus granulosus taenia, which passes through the portal system and is stopped in the liver and lungs in 80% of cases. Muscle contractility and lactic acid production prevent the parasite from developing **[69]**. The proximal muscles of the lower limbs are the most commonly parasitised **[74]**. The low contractility and high blood flow of muscle fibres in the roots of the limbs favour the growth of the parasite. Our results are in good agreement with previous studies. The isolated and primitive nature of the muscular hydatid cyst is a property reported in the majority of published series **[69]** and in the 3 cases in our series. The frequency of association with other sites was estimated at 8% **[81]**, which was the case in two of our observations, where muscle hydatidosis was associated with bone hydatidosis. Bone localisation is equally rare, accounting for 0.5 to 2% of cases. The cyst can hardly take on its typical spherical shape in bone, due to the rigid nature of the latter **[82]**. Bone tissue is contaminated by the haematogenous route, after crossing the liver and lung barriers **[8]**. However, in some cases, primary muscle involvement may be the cause of secondary bone invasion **[82]**. This was observed in two of our patients. Involvement of the pelvic girdle is exceptional **[83]**. The iliac bone is involved in 16.4% of cases **[61]**. In our series, only two patients had hydatidosis of the pelvis.In all cases of parasitic disease, a blood count should be taken to check for hypereosinophilia. However, this is not specific **[50]**. In our series, none of the patients showed an increase in eosinophils. Diagnosis of hydatid cysts is based on medical imaging modalities such as radiography, ultrasound, MRI and CT, in order to identify them in the tissues **[84]**. Standard radiography remains the basic examination for the diagnosis of bone hydatidosis. Ultrasound can be used to explore soft tissues, including muscles. Like chest X-rays, ultrasound helps to orientate the diagnosis by looking for other associated visceral disorders **[61]**. Hydatid serology is usually negative, and is generally positive only in cases of infection or rupture of the cyst **[8,60]**. In our series, the result was negative in 3 out of 5 patients. Progression of the disease is extremely slow; most hydatidosis cases are acquired in childhood but generally become symptomatic in adulthood **[50,85]**, as observed in our series. Bone hydatidosis usually affects adult males **[6]**. This is consistent with our results, with bone involvement in two men. However, there was no gender predominance in muscle involvement **[69]**. We noted a slight male predilection in our series (3 men/2 women), which was an inconclusive result due to the small number of patients.The majority of bone hydatidosis cases are asymptomatic. There are no specific symptoms, so complications are generally the reason for detection **[86]**. This is also the case for muscle hydatidosis, where the clinical signs are not specific and the onset is often silent, presenting as a painless, well-limited swelling of soft consistency, with good general condition **[81].** As was the case in our patients.Recurrence is a frequent phenomenon that can occur in bone and muscle hydatidosis. In the case of bone involvement, this recurrence is caused by the infiltration of small vesicles and the absence of a clear delineation between healthy and pathological tissue. This makes radical surgical resection difficult. Furthermore, in the case of muscle involvement, recurrence is less frequent when surgical removal is combined with antihelminthic treatment, which is considered to be the preferred treatment **[60,87].** This finding is illustrated in our results, with 80% of cases relapsing.The use of Benzimidazole derivatives such as Albendazole or Mebendazole prior to surgery is considered adjuvant therapy, in order to reduce the risk of recurrence. None of our patients received antihelminthic treatment, which may explain the high rate of recurrence. Therapeutic follow-up is a major means of detecting possible recurrences, progression or sequelae **[85,87].**

CHAPTER V
CONCLUSION

The results obtained during our study revealed the following: Hydatid cysts can affect different body systems. The liver and lungs are usually the site of the parasite. The location of hydatids in muscle and bone tissue is rare but possible. Within the muscle, the production of lactic acid and permanent muscle contractions make it more difficult for the scolex to nidate, making it an unfavourable environment for the parasite's larval development.The clinical appearance of the disease is characterised by an insidious and asymptomatic onset, often revealed by pain and swelling.The disease affects both sexes, and appears to be more common in adults, with an average age of 35.80 years. Bone involvement is widespread in males, as is muscular hydatidosis, where a slight male predominance was recorded in this series of studies. However, the small number of patients makes the results inconclusive on this point, underlining the importance of conducting further research, while increasing the sample size, to better define the epidemiological characteristics of this parasitosis. Primary muscle involvement was the most common in this study (60%), but our results also showed that secondary bone invasion is possible (40%).Early diagnosis of the disease relies mainly on medical imaging data, which can also be used to establish a pre-operative map and detect any recurrence. Biological tests also play a valuable role in the diagnosis and monitoring of patients. Surgery is the treatment of choice, providing a cure on its own. Nevertheless, a combination with medical treatment, particularly antihelminthic drugs, could offer better management in terms of controlling the incidence of recurrence, as demonstrated by the present study, in which 80% of the cases studied had recurrent cysts, underlining the importance of conducting further research to assess the efficacy of adjuvant treatment with Benzimidazole derivatives and to define the risk factors for recurrence. Despite therapies that have produced satisfactory results, the fight against this parasite is still essentially based on preventive measures aimed at interrupting the parasite cycle, avoiding the dissemination of eggs by the definitive host:

✓ Avoid emotional contact with dogs.

✓ Improving the hygiene of cattle slaughtering, or even eliminating it, especially in highly endemic areas.

✓ Vaccination of sheep with a recombinant antigen (EG95), which provides an effective tool for eradicating the disease.

✓ Raise public awareness of the risks associated with the practice of ritual sacrifice, by mobilising appropriate preventive measures.

BIBLIOGRAPHY

[1]. Wejih D., Ramzi N., Karim A., Chadli D. Le cyst hydatique du foie. Revue Francophone des Laboratoires. 2017 ; 2017(491) :31-7.

[2]. El Biaze M. Thoracic hydatidosis: news and developments. Revue des maladies respiratoires. 2006 ; 23(4) :80-2.

[3]. Tliba S., Boudraa R., Fadla H., Mansour A., Samai N., Houam K., et al. Hydatid cysts of the orbit. Journal de Neurochirurgie; 2008.

[4]. Belamalem S., Khadmaoui A., Hami H., Harrak M., Aujjar N., Mokhtari A., et al. Epidemiology of hydatidosis in the Gharb Region (Chrarda Beni Hssen) Morocco. Evolution. 2014 ; 161 :100.

[5]. Rezig AL. Hydatidosis of the bone. Revue du Rhumatisme. 2002 ; **69**(8) :835-841.

[6]. Benrami M., Bouklata S., Asefsa Z., Hammani L., Imani F. Hydatid cyst of the sternum: a rare localization. Journal de Radiologie. 2007 ; **88**(2) :277-9.

[7]. Rafiqi K., Rafaoui A., Sirrajelhak M., Messoudi A., Abouali HA., Rafai M., et al. Primary hydatid cyst of the thigh in a bodybuilder. A case report and review of the literature. Journal of Sports Traumatology. 2016 ; 33(2) :107-9.

[8]. Loudiye H., Aktaou S., Hassikou H., El Bardouni A., El Manouar M., Fizazi M., et al. Hydatidosis of the bone: study of 11 cases. Revue du Rhumatisme. 2003 ; 70(9) :732-5.

[9]. Moor L. and Dalley AF.. Anatomie clinique.2 éd. Bruxelle : Deboeck Editions ; 2007.

[10]. Pastoureau P. Physiology of bone tissue development. INRAE Productions Animales. 1990;3(4):265-73.

[11]. Marie P. Physiology of bone tissue. Immuno-analysis & Specialized Biology. 1992;7(6):17-24.

[12]. Massart C., Guggenbuhl P., Souberbielle JC. Mode o f action of calciotropic hormones. Revue du Rhumatisme Monographies. Sept 2012;79(4):210-4

[13]. Hammoudi SS. Le cours d'anatomie- Appareil locomoteur 1. Membre supérieur. 2e ed. Algiers: Auto-edition; 2004.

[14]. Michel Lacombe. Précis d'anatomie et de physiologie humaines. 28e ed. Rueil-Malmaison; 2000.

[15]. da Silva AM. From "hydatid cyst" to cystic echinococcosis: the impact of history in nomenclature. E-Mem Acad Natle Chir. 2017;16(3):007.

[16]. QASRI MM. Imaging of complicated hepatic hydatid cyst. Marrakech: Faculty of medicine and pharmacy; 2019.

[17]. McManus DP. Current status of the genetics and molecular taxonomy of Echinococcus species. Parasitology. 2013;140(13):1617-23.

[18]. Madani R., Shemshadi B., Sh RB. Genetic Affinity of Echinococcus granulosus protoscolex in Human and Sheep in East Azerbaijan, Iran. Archives of Razi Institute. 2020;75(1):47.

[19]. Elissondo MC., Dopchiz MC., Zanini F., Perez H., Brasesco M., Denegri G. Strain characterization of Echinococcus granulosus protoscoleces of cattle origin using the in vitro vesicular development. Parasite. 2005;12(2):159-64.

[20]. Romig T., Ebi D., Wassermann M. Taxonomy and molecular epidemiology of Echinococcus granulosus sensu lato. Veterinary parasitology. 2015;213(3-4):76-84.

[21]. Muqaddas H., Mehmood N., Arshad M. Genetic variability and diversity of Echinococcus granulosus sensu lato in human isolates of Pakistan based on cox1 mt-DNA sequences (366bp). Acta tropica. 2020;207:105470.

[22]. Klotz F., Nicolas X., Debonne JM., Garcia JF., Andreu JM. Hydatid cysts of the liver. Encycl Méd Chir. 2000.

[23]. Yennek S.,Yennek S. Retrospective study on hydatid cyst in the Dellys region. Tizi-Ouzou: Université Mouloud Mammeri; 2017.

[24]. Eckert J, Gemmell MA, Meslin FX, Pawlowski ZS, Organization WH. WHO/OIE manual on echinococcosis in humans and animals: a public health problem of global concern. World Organisation for Animal Health; 2001. 262 p.

[25]. Thompson RCA. Chapter Two - Biology and Systematics of Echinococcus. In: Thompson RCA, Deplazes P, Lymbery AJ. Advances in Parasitology. Academic Press; 2017. p. 65-109.

[26]. Vallat B., Edwards S. Manual of diagnostic tests and vaccines for terrestrial animals (mammals, birds and bees). World Organisation for Animal Health, 2009.

[27]. Sayeh I. and Chekkal I. Study of hydatid cysts in sheep, cattle and goats in abattoirs in the Biskra region. Biskra: Université Mohamed Khider; 2021.

[28]. Aubry P. Hydatidosis or hydatid cyst. Centre René Labusquière, Institut de Médecine Tropicale, Université de Bordeaux, 33076 Bordeaux (France); 2022. Available at: http //www.medecinetropicale.com

[29]. Bronstein JA, Klotz F. Larval cestodoses. EMC-Maladies infectieuses. 2005;2(2):59-83.

[30]. Ketata H., Peyromaure M. Hydatid cyst of the kidney. In: Annales d'urologie. Elsevier; 2004. p. 259-65.

[31]. Bellili K. and Bendou G. Hydatid cyst research on sheep, cattle and goats in the few slaughterhouses of the Tizi-Ouzou region. Tizi-Ouzzou: Université Mouloud Mammeri; 2018.

[32]. Woolsey ID, Miller AL. Echinococcus granulosus sensu lato and Echinococcus multilocularis: A review. Research in veterinary science. 2021;135(Journal Article):517-22.

[33]. Mandal S., Mandal MD. Human cystic echinococcosis: epidemiologic, zoonotic, clinical, diagnostic and therapeutic aspects. Asian Pac J Trop Med. 2012;5(4):253-60.

[34]. Sanchez L., Mayta H., Jara LM., Verástegui M., Gilman RH., Gómez-Puerta LA., et al. Echinococcus granulosus sensu stricto and E. canadensis are distributed in livestock of highly endemic area in the Peruvian highlands. Acta Tropica. 2022;225:106178.

[35]. Grosso G., Gruttadauria S., Biondi A., Marventano S., Mistretta A. Worldwide epidemiology of liver hydatidosis including the Mediterranean area. World J Gastroenterol.2012;18(13):1425-37

[36]. Bardonnet K., Benchikh-Elfegoun MC., Bart JM., Harraga S., Hannache N., Haddad S., et al. Cystic echinococcosis in Algeria: cattle act as reservoirs of a sheep strain and may contribute to human contamination. Vet Parasitol. 2003;116(1):35-44.

[37]. Kayouèche F., Chassagne M., Benmakhlouf A., Abrial D., Dorr N., Benlatreche C., et al. Socio-ecological factors associated with the risk of familial hydatidosis in the wilaya of Constantine (Algeria) through interviews with households living in urban and rural areas. Journal of veterinary medicine. 2009;160(3):119-26.

[38]. Gessese AT. Review on Epidemiology and Public Health Significance of Hydatidosis. Lobetti R, editor. Veterinary Medicine International. 2020;2020:1-8.

[39]. Ripoche M. 2009. The fight against hydatidosis in Sardinia. Doctor of Veterinary Medicine thesis. Toulouse National Veterinary School, 108pp.

[40]. Tourne M., Dupin C., Mordant P., Neuville M., Taillé C., Danel C. Native pulmonary hydatid cyst. Annales de Pathologie. 2019;39(1):47-53.

[41]. Derfoufi O., Ngoh Akwa E., Elmaataoui A., Miss E., Esselmani H., Lyagoubi M., et al. Epidemiological profile of hydatidosis in Morocco from 1980 to 2008. In: Annales de biologie clinique. 2012. p. 457.

[42]. Brehm K., Koziol U. Echinococcus-host interactions at cellular and molecular levels. Advances in parasitology. 2017;95:147-212.

[43]. Ghadhoune H., Chaari A., Baccouche N., Chelly H., Bouaziz M. Ischaemic stroke: a rare complication of liver hydatid cyst. Annales Françaises d'Anesthésie et de Réanimation. 2013 ; 32(10) :715-7.

[44]. Sakhri J., Ben Ali A. The hydatid cyst of the liver. Journal de Chirurgie 2004; 141(6):381-9.

[45]. El Khattabi W., Aichane A., Riah A., Jabri H., Afif H., Bouayad Z. Analysis of the radioclinical semiology of pulmonary hydatid cyst. Revue de Pneumologie Clinique. 2012 ; 68(6) :329-37.

[46]. Bounaim A., Zentar A., Ait Ali A., El Kaoui H., Sair K. Primary hydatid cyst of the spleen: two cases. Can we be conservative? J Afr Hepato Gastroenterol. 2009 ; 3(1) :46-8.

[47]. Hafsa C., Belguith M., Golli M., Rachdi H., Kriaa S., Elamri A., et al. Imaging of hydatid cyst of the lung in children. Journal de Radiologie. Apr 2005; 86(4):405-10.

[48]. Bouchikh M., Ouadnouni Y., Msougar Y., Lakrambi M., Smahi M., Harrak L., et

al. Hydatid cyst of the lung revealed by dysphonia. Revue des Maladies Respiratoires. 1 sept 2007 ; 24(7) :905-8.

[49]. Jellali MA., Zrig M., Zrig A., Mnif H., Hmida B., Abid A., et al. Pathological humeral fracture revealing a hydatid bone cyst. Médecine et Maladies Infectieuses. March 2011 ; 41(3) :164-6.

[50]. Mseddi M., Mtaoumi M., Dahmene J., Ben Hamida R., Siala A., Moula T., et al. Muscular hydatid cyst. Revue de Chirurgie Orthopédique et Réparatrice de l'Appareil Moteur. May 2005 ; 91(3) :267-71.

[51]. Djenna Z., Tobbi A., Abdeslam S. Multiple cerebral hydatidosis operated on in a single stage. Neurosurgery. 2020 ; 66(4) :291.

[52]. Roux FX, Sainte-Rose C, Pierre-Kahn A, Renier D, Hirsch JF. Cerebral hydatid cysts in children. Médecine et Maladies Infectieuses. 1985 ; 15(10) :541-6.

[53]. Jouhadi Z., Ailal F., Dreoua N., Zine Eddine A., Abid A., Skalli A., et al. Cardiac hydatid cyst. La Presse Médicale. 2004 ; 33(18) :1260-3.

[54]. Fadil A., Ait Bolbarod A., El Fares F. Hydatid cyst of the pancreas. A case report. Annales de Chirurgie. 2000 ; 125(2) :173-5.

[55]. El Mansari O., Zentar A., Sair K., Sakit F., Bounaim A., Janati IM. Peritoneal hydatidosis. About 12 cases. Annales de Chirurgie. 2000 ; 125(4) :353-7.

[56]. Bhutani N., Kajal P. Hepatic echinococcosis: A review. Ann Med Surg (Lond). 2018;36:99-105.

[57]. Eckert J., Deplazes P. Biological, Epidemiological, and Clinical Aspects of Echinococcosis, a Zoonosis of Increasing Concern. Clin Microbiol Rev. 2004 ;17(1):107-35.

[58]. Sakhri J., Ben Ali A. The hydatid cyst of the liver. Journal de Chirurgie. 2004;141(6):381-9.

[59]. Gottstein B., Reichen J. Hydatid lung disease (echinococcosis/hydatidosis). Clinics in Chest Medicine. 2002;23(2):397-408.

[60]. Jerbi OS., Abid F., Mnif H., et al. Primary hydatid cyst of the thigh. A rare localization. Revue de Chirurgie Orthopédique et Traumatologique. 2010;96(1):105-8.

[61]. Nhamoucha Y., Alaoui O., Doumbia A., et al. A bony hydatid cyst: a rare location in the iliac bone. Pan Afr Med J. 2016.

[62]. Moujahid M., Tajdine MT., Achour A., Janati MI. Hydatid cyst of the spleen. About 36 cases. Experience of the department. J Afr Hepato Gastroenterol. 2009;3(4):212-5.

[63]. Ousadden A., Raiss M., Hrora A., AitLaalim S., Alaoui M., Sabbah F., et al. Hydatid cysts of the spleen: radical or conservative surgery? Pan Afr Med J. 2010;5:21.

[64]. Bakkali A., Jaabari I., Bouhdadi H., Razine R., Bennani Mechita N., El Harrag J., et al. Cardiac hydatid cysts: 17 cases operated. Annals of Cardiology and Aneiology. 2018;67(2):67-73.

[65]. Fekak H., Bennani S., Rabii R., Mezzour MH., Debbagh A., Joual A., et al. Hydatid cyst of the kidney: about 90 cases. Annales d'Urologie. 2003;37(3):85-9.

[66]. Bourée P., Lançon A. Diagnosis of blood hypereosinophilia. Revue Française des Laboratoires. March 2000; 2000(321) :67-71.

[67]. Zait H., Boulahbel M., Normand AC., Zait F., Achir I., Guerchani MK, et al. Parasitological study of 78 cases of human cystic echinococcosis collected between 2005 and 2012 at the CHU Mustapha in Algiers. Pathology Biology. 2014 ; 62(6) :369-76.

[68]. Ben Khalfallah A., Ben Slima H. Hydatid cyst of the heart. Which imaging modality for an accurate diagnosis? Annals of Cardiology and Aneiology. 2017 ; 66(2) :102-8.

[69]. Alouini Mekki R., Mhiri Souei M., Allani M., Bahri M., Arifa N., Jemni Gharbi H., et al. Soft tissue hydatid cyst: contribution of MRI (About three observations). Journal de Radiologie. 2005 ; 86(4) :421-5.

[70]. Noomen F., Mahmoudi A., Fodha M., Boudokhane M., Hamdi A., Fodha M. 40-775 Surgical treatment of hydatid cysts of the liver. EMC - Surgery. 2013 ; 8.

[71]. Bentani N., Basraoui D., Wakrim B., Hiroual MR., Cherif Idrissi Ganouni N., Dahami .Z., et al. Hydatid cyst of the kidney: radiological and therapeutic aspects. Progrès en Urologie. 2012 ; 22(16) :999-1003.

[72]. Bedioui H., Nouira K., Daghfous A., Ammous A., Ayari H., Rebai W. et al. Primary hydatid cyst of the psoas: 9 Tunisian cases and review of the literature. Med Trop. 2008; 68: 261-266.

[73]. Buttenschoen K., Carli Buttenschoen D. Echinococcus granulosus infection: the challenge of surgical treatment. Langenbeck's Archives of Surgery. 2003 ;388(4) :218-30.

[74]. Hamouda O., Benchikh M., Boudjouraf N. Hydatid cyst of the psoas: about a case. Batna J Med Sci. 2015;2(1):82-84.

[75]. Orhan G., Ozay B., Tartan Z., et al. Surgery of cardiac hydatid cysts. Thirty-nine years of experience. Annals of Cardiology and Aneology. 2008 ;57(1) :58-61.

[76]. Tlili-Graiess K., El-Ouni F., Gharbi-Jemni H., et al. Cerebral hydatidosis. Journal of Neuroradiology. 2006;33(5):304-18.

[77]. Stamatakos M., Sargedi C., Stefanaki C., Safioleas C., Matthaiopoulou I., Safioleas M. Anthelminthic treatment: An adjuvant therapeutic strategy against Echinococcus granulosus. Parasitology International. 2009;58(2):115-20.

[78]. Gauci C., Heath D., Chow C., Lightowlers MW. Hydatid disease: vaccinology and development of the EG95 recombinant vaccine. Expert Review of Vaccines. 2005;4(1):103-12.

[79]. Campoy E., Rodriguez-moreno J., Del Blanco J., Narvaez J., Clavaguera T., Roig-escofet D. Hydatid disease an unusual cause of chronic monarthritis. Arthritis & Rheumatism. 1995;38(9):1338-9.

[80]. Laatamna A., Bouragba M., Reghaissia N., Benhadj N., Mahdjoub I., Harfouche K., Bouragba N., et al. Epidemiological profile and fertility assessment of hydatid cysts surgically removed from patients in Djelfa province, Algeria. Annals of Parasitology. 2021 ;67(2), 337- 340.

[81]. Benhaddou H., Margi M., Kissra M., Benhmamouche MN. Hydatid cyst of the trapezius muscle: an unusual localization. Archives de Pédiatrie. March 2010;17(3):263-5.

[82]. Polat P., Kantarci M., Alper F., Suma S., Koruyucu MB., Okur A. Hydatid Disease from Head to Toe. RadioGraphics 2003; 23:475-494.

[83]. Bennani J. Rare localization of hydatid cyst: a case report. Revue Neurologique. 2016; 172, A129.

[84]. Combalia A., Sastre S. Hydatid cyst of the gluteal muscle. Two cases. Revue de la littérature. Revue du Rhumatisme. 2005;72(9):851-853.

[85]. Inayat F., Rana RE., Azam S., Ahmad R., Ahmad S. Pelvic bone hydatidosis: a dangerous crippling disease. Cureus. 2019;11(4).

[86]. Zlitni M., Ezzaouia K., Lebib H., Karray M., Kooli M., Mestiri M. Hydatid Cyst of Bone: Diagnosis and Treatment. World J. Surg. 2001;(25) 75-82.

[87]. Arazi M., Erikoglu M., Odev K., Memik R., Ozdemir M. Primary Echinococcus Infestation of the Bone and Muscles. Clinical Orthopaedics and Related Research. 2005;(432)234-241.

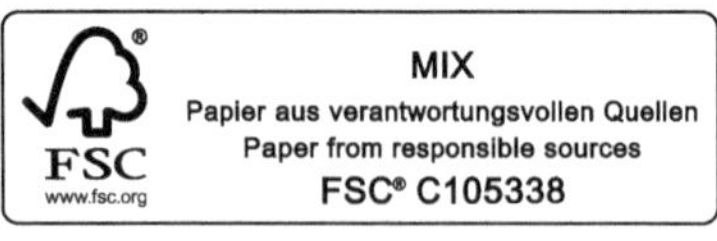

Printed by Books on Demand GmbH, Norderstedt / Germany